OF SEA

Elizabeth-Jane Burnett is an author, academic and founder of *Grow Your Own Creativity*. A writer of English and Kenyan heritage, she was born in Devon and her work is inspired by the landscape in which she was raised. Her poetry has been highly commended in the Forward Prize and *Swims* was longlisted for the Laurel Prize and a Sunday Times Poetry Book of the Year. She was selected for the 2020 British Council/National Centre for Writing International Literature Showcase and leads the British Academy/Leverhulme Trust project, *Creative Writing and Climate Change: Moss, Wetlands and Women* (2018-20).

ALSO BY ELIZABETH-JANE BURNETT

POETRY

Swims (Penned in the Margins, 2017)

CRITICAL

A Social Biography of Contemporary Innovative Poetry Communities: The Gift, the Wager and Poethics (Palgrave, 2017)

NON-FICTION

The Grassling (Allen Lane, 2019)

Of Sea

ELIZABETH-JANE BURNETT

Penned in the Margins

LONDON

PUBLISHED BY PENNED IN THE MARGINS
Toynbee Studios, 28 Commercial Street, London E1 6AB
www.pennedinthemargins.co.uk

First published 2021

Printed in the United Kingdom by TJ Books Limited

ISBN
978-1-908058-82-9

CONTENTS

INTERMISSION: CALL OF THE SEA

ABOVE

NOTE ON THE TEXT

A recent survey for a site at Dawlish Warren in Devon shows the presence of 39 invertebrates. The poems chart encounters through swimming.

Of Sea

SUN

Prickly Cockle

A sunrise in a shell.
How you start light,
then take flight down
your own body, shedding
fire. I happen upon you
as daylight, dizzy with
waking, all efforts
of not breaking exposed,
glazed open. I would
no more touch than break
you. I would no more break
than touch you. A hair,
a line is all it takes.

Great Green Bush Cricket

All a-glow

the green   a-gleam

a-glass   a-gasp

a-grasp   the grassy sea.

Dip up   the freshly

of a crackle a-field.

a wing   that sings

a-clatter   a-chatter

the branch   of wave

cut water   lie low

Barrel Jellyfish

'The [US] administration has taken a hatchet to climate change language across government websites ... mentions of climate change have been excised, buried or stripped of any importance'
The Guardian, 14th May, 2017

To be a risky thing, run in water thing, early riser.

As a robin, as a jaybird, as an eye. We put our parts together. We outward

form. We resemble. As rusks, as plants grow in marshy ground, as wind. We be longing to peril, in press of pressing on. If we disappear

try us with different titles.

Say we were frost or fruit. Say we were whale fat. Say we were good for the economy, or don't say anything.

Plait a rope, thread a hundred of our mouths together, let only sea unravel us.

Look for us, even after we are gone. With eight arms there's a chance one may keep, wrongly filed under

weapons.

White-tailed Bumble Bee

go
just
pack
flowers

go
just
pack
flowers

go
just
pack
flowers

go
just
pack
flowers

go
just
pack
flowers

go
just
pack
flowers

go
just   go
pack   just   go
flowers   pack   just
flowers   flowers   pack
                                flowers

do you ever go
to sea just pack
up & leave all flowers
at the shore?

go   go   go   go
just   just   just   just
pack   pack   pack   pack
flowersflowersflowersflowers

Small Blue

for Olly Watts

'The S-shaped butterfly banks ... were primarily designed to spread the range of the small blue butterfly ... To do this we have planted or sown seed of the butterfly caterpillar food plants that thrive on thin chalk soils'
— Patrick Cashman, RSPB, 2018

                        small blue   small blue

            small blue   small blue   small blue   small blue

small blue   small blue   small blue   small blue   small blue

dark green fritillary

dark green fritillary

common blue

marbled white

marsh fritillary

            Devil's-bit scabious

            horseshoe vetch horseshoe vetch

                        squinancywort   squinancywort

                        mouse-ear hawkweed   mouse-ear hawkweed

                                    wild thyme   wild thyme

                                                carline thistle

                                    rockrose   rockrose

                        carline thistle   carline

                        violet   hairy violet hairy

            hairy violet hairy violet   hairy violet

kidney vetch kidney vetch kidney vetch kidney vetch

kidney vetch kidney vetch kidney vetch kidney

kidney vetch kidney vetch

Squat Furrow Bee

Between   a basket,   a gland,
an abdomen,   a hive,
a neck,   a belly,
a barrier,   a square,
a muscle,   a hollow,   a shell
          pulls between us,   bearing
legs,   bearing wings,
a spinning causeway of wicker   work.

MOON

Ragworm

In the new sand, in the new tide, in the blossom
of a new stride, ragworms start to shimmy.
In the moon tide, in the moon dune, in the blossom
of a new moon, ragworms flexy shiver.
What is it that makes them sway, half-dizzy with the dance
of day, and sink into the frothy night all silver from the milky light
and all the mud-life springing, to see the ragworms swimming?
In the not-sea, in the not-land, in the mizzle
of the wet sand, all our questions crumble.
All our lines break, all that's fixed shakes, when we nestle
in the worms' wake, all our meanings fumble,
unable to take hold of us. We shimmer in the night's impulse
too quick for any tight embrace, all slippy through the waterlace,
and all the mud-life springing, in all the love of being.

Mud Shrimp

she swam
only at night
on the spring tides

in the silk light of water
slipping her over
the mud flats

when they studied why she did it
drifted far beyond her limits
though it made her vulnerable
to prey

several theories came
but none swam
at night in a spring tide
in the silk light unsure
of itself
becoming only what is left
after breaking

Sea Mouse

stomach of fur
coughed up at low tide
stranded

snowfall of fur
dusting the mouth
sanded

out of this
worms fall soft as whispers
coiling

into fauning
"Aphrodita"

& out of her hair come the corpses
of a swallowed sea

Lupin Aphid

As frozen dew the coat of you dusts light,
a brief touch, a whisper of wax
on a body just the colour of the sea.

You live your whole life in one flower.
This, the furthest out you've ever been.
Banished, perhaps, by wolves, by leaves,

by howling roots that tire of the ground.
But every time they take you back: the roots,
the wolves, the leaves; as if they know they moonless go
who go without your sheen.

Ghost Moth

salt	wings
marsh	over
shallow	grass
soil	salt
shingle	marsh
marram	silver
grass	path
fescue	of
grass	pollen
tidal	flight
path	of
creek	swollen
of	night
pollen	calls
falls	flings
in whispers	

Silver-stiletto Fly

Of moon, of sea, of hair
of colour, of tongue, of scale
of waves, of fox, of coin
of light, of leaf.

As quick, as fish, as spoon,
as work, as thread, as an apricot
keen, alive, a line,
a lilt.

BELOW

Murky-legged Legionnaire Fly

Muscles
    move
the murk
    of sea-dirt
        blurt of sun
        off-wing or throat
   floats for a blink
then dark flickerless mud
along the mouth
darkness in the teeth
a suck of salt too steep
for breath to follow
only seconds from
defeat the water
darkling deep.

Millipede

Maw.
Lick, mulch, moss.
Find a way in by skin.
I tear! I burst! Cut off
the fruit of my teeth,
a drum, & bone.
Find a way out of skin.
Bite. Wear away at.
Nag, gnat, gnaw,
flow, earth nymph,
soil swimmer, flow,
polish, the clear part
of any stone.

Green Leaf Worm

Turn, curve, slink
through sheet
of water.
I sting.
I pierce men.
A constellation
of shark's teeth.
Strapless.
Wingless.
An unforgettable pop
song. A wind
flows through me.
Limbless.
All I do is echo.

Bootlace Worm

Body within body, whirligig.
Flighty.
If 180 ft long,
you must have a system.
You must know
a helicopter
or a tuning peg.
Or, if washed ashore,
how to be
a sea shell.
But these get lost
in the twirling muscle
of the present
& the scream of being
one thing.

Earwig

By worm, by wagon, by wheel,
by wiggle, by wing of skin.
Molt five times before settling.
No eel, no deer, no mole,
no seal, no goat's grip or hide.
Fleece Bird. Strip Wind. Bark Blow.
Flay Feather. Cut Flight. Kite.

INTERMISSION:
CALL OF THE SEA

A Chord of Sea

		come	come inside	come in
	ŭka	ŭka thiini	ŭka thiini	ŭka thiini
light	light	light luminous	luminescence	bioluminescence

A Chord of Sands

come wave

ũka haha ũka ava   back   over your

red red come come   back   mountains calling mother there is   a tongũe

home home home

A Chord of Earth

come   wave
        ūka haha ūka ava   back
red red come come   back   mountains calling mother there is
    home home home

Sun, a Sea-olet

Songs are homes that hold us in the swell,
in waltz of whelk, in tiny spirals flung,
they steady us, bright anchors for the cells.
Songs are homes that hold us in the swell
when we lack a centre there are bells
to bring us back, in level beats of sun,
songs are homes that hold us in the swell
in waltz of whelk, in tiny spirals flung.

Echo (a sea-olet)

Songs are homes made on the move, they dwell
in us and we in them, as moons
    guiding the cells
songs are homes made on the move, they dwell
in wings, in limbless shimmerings, in shells
    of dark, of dunes
songs are homes made on the move, they dwell
in us and we in them, as moons.

Seannet

There is a lullaby in all of us.
A call of sea, a song of earth, fluid
fluttering of lungs strung in softness,
body and spirit in endless duet.
Deep-drenched, the invitation in our cells
is stirred by tracks of moon and dunes of sun
burrowing awake in the dark swell —
ũka thinni — *come!* The decision
is made before it's known as every wave
return you to what you have always been —
a body without end, spineless but brave
now you're in, adrift, dripping with dream.
There is a lullaby in all of us,
a language of sea, a fathomless trust.

Song of the Sea

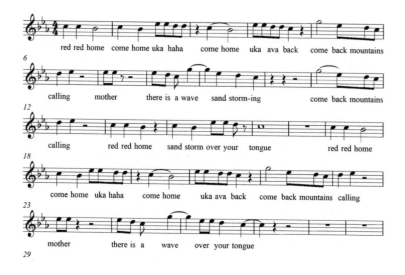

ABOVE

Sand Flea

A hop, a skip, a dancer.
A leap, a lindy, an aviator.
Originating in Harlem,
in Dawlish, in the early rap
lyrics of the high-tide mark.

A beat, a whip of sand, a throb
of heart, a track made by breathing.
Appearing in darkness, night-jigger
or jar. Moth, mite, specked,
missed. The size of the space
between words is

Ruddy Darter

       To throw
yourself against an arrow
       or tide
to startle or stitter
       sharpen, glitter
as mackerel
       leap sudden
stutter water
       breath dug
as a root
       from body ripped
up like a fished
       wing
tip.

Hoverfly

Things pass
over: nerve, wing, a broad
beating sky that never fills
entirely like the sea

in the midst of low
colour, a twist of sky
peels a lemon

causing you to rise
from thick seaweed, pop
through sparkled water

where waves blossom
sun foams
your eyes lift up from
their bones

a whole sky clearing your throat:
such hope.

Brimstone

A simmering
sky, I tuck myself
under.
Nothing can catch
a brink, a bank, an edge,
even if it does flow
over.
I take my body
to the margins.
Hold. Hover.

Gold Swift

Outglimmer, outshimmer, outgleam,
rush, bright gull. Whether bird or
plane or butterfly. Whether dancing girl
or alien. Whether plant or a belonging
to another country. Here is what you are.
Was it air, was it sea, was it land,
was it words, was it paper, was it rot,
was it danger, was it promise, was it done or
was it thrown, was it foretold, was it meant,
was it a scent similar to pineapple
that brought you here is where you are.
Was it bracken. Was it an impediment
to motion. Was it fern or foreign. Was it
rust or was it rush. Is it a game we can all play.
A name? Or instruction.

Gatekeeper

When nothing is full or dirtless.
Not to be eaten or confessed.
When the unwhole, unmooned
surface is left. There will be no
swimming in no sea there will be
no swimming & no sea there will be
no swimming & no clean.

Meadow Brown

I don't know much of abundance
(air-tight, tight-stretched, tight-lipped,
tight-laced, water-tight, close knit,
sleep- skin- sit-)

so when you come in your hundreds,
there is nothing to compare you to.
An excess of blowing? An outrage of wing?
A departure of reason, fluttered fling
beyond the subject. Out of reach of.
Before. Sea-shorn.

Painted Lady

'And swimming my slow breast stroke out to the channel I saw a darkwinged butterfly come flying in above the waves, moving with the breeze, heading for the dunes. Was this a migrant painted lady, third generation, from Africa?'
— Tony Lopez

found
tips
sound
sedge
elk
rune
chimes
chinks
wet
held
light parts blades, parts wings, parts limbs unhinge a falling land

Dusky Sallow

Spit out your dirty yellows, greys, creams,
take them out completely. Hollow. Else find yourself

compared to dead grass, or bronzed, the hue of a statue.
Or find yourself without value, sickly or wan, pallid

or pale. Find that hair, wolves, & waves reflect you
more than your own words. This will happen. Is

happening. Has happened again, is about to.
I don't know what more to do than strike

out into what I love, over & under & over & out into
what I love, under & over & under & over & out into
what I love is the freshness, eagerness, insolence
of sea. How it picks itself up without looking.

SURFACING

Sand Crab

In the clay in the loam in the top of the soil
in the sand in the molt of the sea

in the light sand the light sound of shift in the swash
zone waves break burrowing for release

in the bend of the body
I balance my current only takes me back
when seawards seawards is the call of my curve
& no turning.

Spider Crab

Posterior
rapid, with horses
post-human, belonging to
post-nature, the powers of the body
post-political, intending to live in a city
post-landscape, to plant trees
post-anthropocene, no matching terms for
post-lyrical, a song, a dance
post-fact, anything done with legs
is only part of it.

Ground Beetle

To be sung/clicked/slicked

Some beetles make sounds, usually scraping their mouthparts together or rubbing their legs on their bodies.

ch-ch-ch   ///
ch-ch-ch-ch   ////

how to make such a little   /////
how to make such a little sOund that you /// know I'm talking //
how to make such a little sOund that you /// know I'm talking to you

when I   //   ch-ch-ch   ///   when I   //   ch-ch //
know I'm overwHELMing ch-ch-ch ////

every sound ///   every nON-sound   ///   I want to pluck out my teeth & pLA
LA LA LAnt them // under your // pilla-o-a   // under your pillo-a-so you know
I'm talking // ch-ch-ch /// talking with such a little sound //

I pLA LA LAnt a little   sand   sound

                             sound sand

you know I'm such a little sound sand

                             sand   sound

I pLA LA LAnt a little   sand   sound

                             sound sand

you know I'm such a little   sound sand

                             sand   sound

talking with such a lit-tt-tt ch-ch-ch   lit-tt-tt ch-ch-ch   tt-tt-tt tt-tt-tt tt-tt-tt
tt-tt-ttle sound /////

cl-cl-cl   ///
cl-cl-cl-cl-cl-cl   //////

how to hear such a brittle
how to hear such a brittle sOund that you /// know I'm listening
how to hear such a brittle sOund that you /// know I'm bristling when you

cl-cl-cl   ///   when you   //   cl-cl-cl   // know I'm listening to you

every move // every nON-move // I want to pull out my legs and swi-wiwi-
WING them over my ears & nobody hears them over my ears & nobody hears when

I sWI-WI-WI-WING a little   sand   sound
                                   sound sand

you know we're such a little   sound sand
                                   sand   sound

we sWI-WI-WI-WING a little   sand   sound
                                   sound sand & it feels like talking   /////

t-t-t   ///

tt-tt-tt-tt-tt ch-ch-ch-ch-ch   ch-ch-ch-ch-ch-ch
                                tck-tck-tck   ///   tck-tck-tck tck-tck-tck
cl-cl-cl-cl-cl ch-ch-ch   cl-cl-cl-ch-ch-ch
///   tck-tck-tck   tck-tck-tck
          ch-ch-ch   ch-ch-ch   s-s-s-s-s s-s-s-s-s s-s-s-s-ss-s

s-WI-WI-WI-WI-WING   p-LA-LA-LA-LA-LA
                     s-WI-WI-WI-WI-WING p-LA-LA-LA-LA-LA

s-WI-WI-WI-WI-WING   p-LA-LA-LA-LA-LA
                     s-WI-WI-WI-WI-WING   p-LA-LA-LA-LA   LA

Paignton Cockle

Shell doesn't cover
you. Nor sky, nor sea,
nor sand. Your lift
of land. Your froth of
stone. Your pearl,
your peal of sound.

Bell doesn't cover
it. The chink of tide
that worries you.
The chime of colour
coming into view:
scarlet, wax, star.

I run my tongue
along you. I could
wash you clean,
mother of harlots
& abominations.

Or lie you
on your back so you

don't show. Berry,
fever, seal. Oak,
notch, cloth. The shock
of you all hidden.

Surf Clam

Sometimes it's hard
to be a surfer,
giving all your love
to just one clam.
You'll have bad tides
& he'll have good tides
reaching the high water mark on land.
But if you love him you'll forgive him
even though he's hard to understand
& if you love him, o, be proud of him
cause after all he's just a clam.

STAND BY YOUR CLAM
GIVE HIM TWO VALVES TO CLING TO
& SOMETHING WARM TO COME TO
WHEN SANDS ARE COLD & LONELY
STAND BY YOUR CLAM
& SHOW THE WORLD YOU LOVE HIM
KEEP GIVING ALL THE LOVE YOU CAN
STAND BY YOUR CLAM

Sea Anemone

she
    windblown sand
    seashell sand
    shifting sand
she
    sea sandwort
    sea rocket
    sea holly
she
    half sand
she both sea
    she half sea
she both sand

she is a both-formed thing

she
    wool sand
    cotton sand
    wood sand
she
    sea leather
    sea crystal
    sea skin
she
half wool
she both skin
she half skin
she both wool

she is a woollen skin

she

    asphalt soil

    nylon soil

    sandy soil

she

    landscape

    escape

    seascape

she half soil

she both scape

she half scape

she both soil

        she escapes

SPILLING

Mud Snail

for Tony Lopez

drifter   on the surface
upside   down dead
                       water

                 floater   upper   sheltered
                  on the littoral fringe
                             lower   very sheltered

                    swimmer upward   of hundreds   of thousands
                                  of hundreds   of thousands
of hundreds   of thousands   of hundreds   of thousands   of hundreds
  of thousands of hundreds of thousands of hundreds of
thousands   of hundreds   of thousands   of hundreds   of
thousands   of hundreds   of thousands   of hundreds   of
thousands   of hundreds   of thousands   of hundreds   of
thousands   of hundreds   of houses   of hundreds   of
houses of   of hundreds   of houses   of hundreds   of
houses of   of sands   of houses   of sand   of
houses of   of sands   of hums   of sand   of
hums   of sand   of hum   of sand   of
humming

Common Blue

for a kin-dread spirit

Pages from my journal, an article on the effects of microplastics
on invertebrates, and an exercise for monitoring water pollution
with invertebrate indicator species are plaited into my hair &
transcribed after swimming.

When the sea's is the first water to touch your throat, the
sky's the first to meet your face and despite the remote
location, microplastic fibres make pools within pools as you
dip first your feet, then legs, then torso, shoulders ducking
before brain can say, don't take hygiene precautions.

Swallows continue the loops within loops as you scull
in dark water. You are early today, the only human body
fibres identified in deep-sea water as clouds bulk and hoard
their rain at a concentration of 70.8 a cormorant pulls
across, a common blue between, monitoring below, more
life than you can touch.

This is a fieldwork exercise that involves sampling
water. Flat on your back you rinse through with cold, in an
all-over spearmint flush with invertebrates. Through a front
crawl, the green undermurk ensures students do not eat,

scratch their noses, or rub their eyes trickle through teeth need to wash with appropriate cleansers.

Rain shatters down and you realise you are drifting. You intensify your purpose. Muscles focus and hurl you towards disease-causing chemicals pulling species together examined clean water (mayfly) some pollution (caddis fly) high pollution (blood worms) dismantling sea until it is clean, filtering blood until it's pristine particles pool at your feet, polymers in surface water sweet new bonds between species lift each other protective in shared care aesthetic. A new bind (synthetic).

Rove Beetle

Seaweed Chords

'Within each quadrat, the percentage cover of four constituents was recorded: bare sand, seaweed, driftwood and pebbles... Carabidae were also more likely to be found when more driftwood or seaweed was present. Staphylinidae were associated with seaweed.'

Red gloss   fold cloth   beetle, from bitan, to bite
Irish moss   body-froth   but beetle, not bittle, means light
Wing toss   moth-soft   soft insect

    Wireweed   fire   sea is aflame
    Japanese   fury   body is tamed
    Wing-free   flier   soft flight

       Honeyware   winged kelp   angel of the sand
       Golden-haired   swift help   sweetening land
       Dabberlocks   Badderlocks   sunspots

         Beautiful fan weed   *To actually have the word*   wing-frolics
         Sunset   *beautiful in your name*   bright toni
         Wingswept   *To burst so thoroughly*   To astonish
                     through wet terrain

Orange Ladybird

A Scale of Rock ~ Langstone Rock is eroding as sea level is rising.
Poem reads down from l. 1 to l.18, or up from l.18 to l.1.

sweetheart, small dart, shimmering

shark in miniature, sparks all over its still being

here is a miracle, a desert's memories in minerals

earth's many syllables talking, lifting, not yet calling it off

there are so many forms of being, if tired, why not try another

red lifts us, as no longer driftless, we sing ourselves in

the rock a witness to each new try at life, in brightness reminds us

to fling in survival of the riskiest grasslight pours in your still being

here is a miracle, our many miracles talking, lifting,

not yet calling it off, lilting, all at the same time pulsing, wriggling,

each of us going our separate ways together and in the exposure

the whole country slides, sea rises, we wait for the ice, we try but

ferric oxide washes off sand storms, floods flash, we cry

for our mothers are mountains not sirens, they call with the redness

of earth singing: take out your spine, re-thread a new life

use seaweed cartilage and bone, with grasslight glow through each fold

take what you have, adapt, *ūka ava* (come back), as golden strobes,

as sun-licked microbes and given the level of risk involved in how we evolve

o let us be   let us be   let us be bold

Meadow Grasshopper

52 words for grass

sikuliaq	*made ice*	the new ice appearing on the sea or on rock surfaces
igalaujait	*which looks like windows*	the rime frost that sticks to grasses and other plants
salt grass	*made of sea*	the grass that sticks to the sea or rock or skin surfaces

salt grass	grass that is on the edge	grass with the veins of meat
cotton grass	verge grass	meat grass
soft grass	grass that is holding history	grass cutlets
grass the sun has licked	hurt grass	hind grass
butter grass	grass that is the shape of loss	shorn grass
flat grass	grass that is nearly not grass	grass near water
grass that has been hit	grass you can see the soil through	shallow grass
deep grass	grass that can be landed on	grass that remembers every tread
puffed grass	grass that feels like feathers	grass that forgets
inland grass	grass glimpsed through cloud	grass that forgets
grass that moves as a sea	woollen grass	hallelujah grass
wrinkled grass	grass the swallows sing of	hallelujah

flecked grass   safe grass   grass that is breathing
                                                                               loud
grass that has been holding sweet grass   that bears witness how
its breath
grass where the sun has hit grass that has been gathered in the dents of our bodies,
it slant   such a deep sense of
        bodies that have been held by rain, grass that has cracked again, grass that has
sunk and swayed, you feel it all, each blade.

Fan-bristled Robberfly

Field: past tense of feel: to have felt
like an eel slipping

Slipping, from sleeping: to dream
of being flat like an image or spread
like felt

Felt, from pelt: a hide of buttercups

Whip or stroke the field, use its
diminutive, whippet: a brisk, nimble
woman, trembling

Fieldet: a list of small things
trembling (a dither, a dodder,
a quiver)

Dune Robberfly

Fieldet: small yellow-legged robber fly
black-jeaned t-shirt fly
go at full speed fly
holding breath about to fall fly
float in air fly
actual 'tremble-wing flies'
feel the field slip fly
to have felt like a dream feels
pelts, peals a prayeret
for over
    & ever
& over
    & ever
what then?

GLOSSARY

ũka ava	(*Kiembu*)	come back
ũka haha	(*Kikuyu*)	come back
ũka thiini	(*Kikuyu*)	come in
sikuliaq	(*Inuktuit*)	made ice
igalaujait	(*Inuktuit*)	which looks like windows

ACKNOWLEDGEMENTS

'Mud Shrimp', 'Mud Snail', 'Sand Crab', 'Sea Anemone' and 'Sea Mouse' appeared in *Poetry* (December 2016) as part of a collaboration with Tony Lopez called *Sea Holly*, originally commissioned for the 2016 Enemies/ Singing Apple Press South-West Poetry Tour, curated by Camilla Nelson and Steven Fowler. 'Dune Robberfly' and 'Fan-bristled Robberfly' appeared in the artist book *Field Notes* (as 'Imagined Etymologies' and 'Imagined Taxonomies') made with Rebecca Thomas and exhibited at the 2017 ASLE UKI conference Cross Multi Inter Trans, curated by Harriet Tarlo and Judy Tucker at Sheffield Hallam University. 'Small Blue' appeared in *Magma* 72 (2018) as part of their Climate Change issue, pairing poets with scientists, and 'Goldswift' in *Harper's Bazaar* (February 2019). 'Ground Beetle' was performed on BBC Radio 3 *The Verb*'s programme on Insects (2019) and 'Millipede' on *The Verb*'s Green Memoir programme (2020). 'Ruddy Darter' and 'Hover Fly' featured in the Aerial Literature Festival (2020) and 'Brimstone', 'Gatekeeper' and 'Common Blue' appeared in *Plumwood Mountain*'s Writing the Pause feature, edited by Jonathan Skinner (2020). 'Sun', 'a Sea-olet' and 'Echo (a sea-olet)' appeared in the *Magma* 79 issue on Dwelling (2021), and 'Painted Lady', 'Dusky Sallow' and 'Meadow Brown' in *Wasafiri*'s issue on Water (summer 2021).

My thanks to these journals and venues for these early engagements, to Tony Lopez for our initial collaboration and Mendoza for early reading. Thanks, as ever, to Tom Chivers and the team at Penned in the Margins, and to my family, especially my mother for language discussion and more.